Tips & Methods

For

Weight Loss

By

William kain

Table of Contents

Introduction

Weight loss is the reduction of total body mass brought on by attempts to become more physically fit and healthy or to modify one's look by slimming down. The major therapy for obesity is weight loss, and there is strong evidence that this helps maintain cardiometabolic health in persons with diabetes with a weight loss of 5–15% and prevents progression from pre-diabetes to type 2 diabetes with a weight loss of 7–10%. In those who are overweight or obese, losing weight can lower health risks, improve fitness, and perhaps postpone the onset of diabetes. Those with knee osteoarthritis may have less pain and more mobility thanks to it. Although weight loss can lower hypertension (*high blood pressure),* it is unclear whether this also lessens hypertension-related harm. By changing your lifestyle to burn more calories than you consume, you can lose weight. Weight gain may be caused by *depression, stress, or boredom;* in these situations, people are urged to seek medical attention. According to a 2010 research, dieters who slept through the night shed more than twice as much weight as those who didn't. Despite speculation that supplementation of vitamin D may aid, research does not support this. Long-term, the majority of dieters gain weight back. The UK National Health Service and the Dietary Guidelines for Americans both state that the keys to achieving and maintaining a healthy weight are being mindful of consuming only the number of calories necessary to fulfill your needs and engaging in regular physical activity. Changes in food and lifestyle must also be permanent for weight loss to be long-term. There is evidence that a combination of dieting and exercise produces the best effects and that neither counseling nor exercise alone can cause weight reduction. Dieting alone can cause significant long-term weight loss. Weight loss is the process of lowering body weight via reducing muscle mass, body fat, or both. To better one's health, attractiveness, or general well-being is a frequent ambition for many people. There are numerous reasons why someone might want to lose weight. For instance, being overweight increases the risk of developing conditions like high blood pressure, diabetes, and heart disease. It may also impact one's confidence and sense of self-worth. It is essential to generate a calorie deficit by either cutting back on calories consumed, upping physical activity, or both to lose weight. Making lifestyle adjustments that support a balanced diet and regular exercise is a healthy and long-lasting way to lose weight. It's critical to understand that there is no one-size-fits-all strategy for weight loss. It is essential to speak with a healthcare expert before beginning any weight loss program because every person has specific circumstances and elements that affect their weight.

**Chapter 1
Understanding the maintenance of weight is crucial**

***Maintaining a healthy weight loss is important**

For general health and well-being, it's imperative to maintain a healthy weight. Obesity or being overweight can raise your risk of getting several illnesses, including diabetes, heart disease, stroke, and some types of cancer. Keeping a healthy weight can enhance physical performance and make it easier and more mobile for people to go about their everyday lives. Maintaining a healthy weight is also crucial for mental wellness. Individuals who are unhappy with their weight may struggle with low self-esteem and a poor perception of their bodies, which can result in sadness and anxiety. Due to the higher chance of developing health issues that call for medical attention and treatment, being overweight or obese can be costly. In general, quality of life can be increased by maintaining a healthy weight. It may result in more energy, higher-quality sleep, and an improved sense of self-worth. Maintaining a healthy weight is crucial for sustaining physical function, mental health, financial savings from medical expenses, and improved quality of life.

***Why gaining weight has risks and is bad for your physical and mental health.**

Following a time of weight loss, gaining weight can be risky and detrimental to your physical and mental well-being. Putting on weight gain can make you more likely to get chronic conditions like type 2 diabetes, high blood pressure, heart disease, and several cancers. Your body's metabolism slows down when you lose weight. The metabolic alterations brought on by gaining weight can make it more difficult to shed weight in the future. Putting on weight again might restrict your physical capabilities and make it more difficult for you to carry out regular tasks like carrying groceries or walking up stairs. Putting on weight can negatively affect how you feel about yourself and your body, which can result in despair and worry. Gaining weight can lower your energy levels, make you feel more tired, and make it harder for you to move around. To avoid these detrimental effects, it's crucial to keep a healthy weight. This can be accomplished by adopting a lasting lifestyle shift, regular physical activity, and healthy eating habits.

***Benefits of long-term weight loss**

There are numerous advantages for both physical and mental health associated with sustained weight reduction, which is defined as reducing weight and keeping it off over an extended period. Long-term weight loss can lower the risk of conditions like type 2 diabetes, heart disease, high blood pressure, and several cancers.

Weight loss can help your cardiovascular system by lowering your blood pressure, cholesterol levels, and risk of heart disease.

Being overweight can strain your joints, causing pain and limiting your mobility. These problems can be resolved, and your general mobility will increase, with further weight loss. Reducing weight can help treat sleep apnea and other sleep-related ailments or conditions, improving the quality of your sleep in general. Long-term weight loss can result in higher self-esteem, fewer signs of anxiety and sadness, and better mental health in general. Reducing weight can increase your energy and lessen feelings of exhaustion. An overall reduction in the risk of chronic diseases, an improvement in physical health, and an improvement in your mental and emotional well-being are all ways that sustained weight loss can enhance your quality of life. It's crucial to highlight that healthy lifestyle changes, such as regular exercise and a balanced diet, should be used to lose weight on a long-term basis rather than crash diets or other drastic weight-loss techniques, which can be dangerous to your health.

Chapter 2

Establishing attainable targets for weight maintenance.

***How to set reasonable objectives for weight loss**

Establishing realistic objectives is a crucial first step in losing weight. Here are some pointers to help you establish realistic goals: Establishing precise goals is crucial because it helps you concentrate on what you want to accomplish. Making your objective more clear, such as "I want to lose 10 pounds in the next two months," will help you achieve it. Setting quantifiable objectives enables you to monitor your progress and maintain motivation. Make your objective more specific, such as "I want to consume 3 servings of veggies and 2 servings of fruits per day," rather than just saying "I want to eat healthier. Overly ambitious ambitions can be frustrating and demotivating. Based on your present way of life and habits, make sure the goals you establish are both attainable and practical. You can feel more motivated and successful along the way by breaking your goals down into manageable, smaller steps. For instance, if your objective is to lose 10 pounds, you could divide it into 5 weeks of losing 2 pounds each week. Celebrating your progress's victories can be beneficial.

***Tracking your weight loss progress is crucial.**

Because it keeps you accountable, motivated, and aware of your progress, tracking is essential for weight loss.

It is easier to observe your improvement, no matter how little it may be when you track it. Even when things get challenging, this might keep you inspired to keep working toward your weight loss objectives. You become responsible for yourself when you keep track of your development. You can identify your areas of improvement and weakness and make necessary corrections. You become more conscious of your daily routines, including what you eat, how frequently you exercise, and how much water you consume. Your ability to make better decisions and maintain your weight loss plans is aided by this insight. If necessary, you can modify your diet and exercise regimen. For instance, you can change your food or exercise routine if you realize that you are not losing weight as quickly as you would like to. This will help you achieve your objectives more quickly. You can do this to celebrate your accomplishments, which can be incredibly inspiring. For instance, you can treat yourself to a non-food treat like a massage or new exercise equipment when you meet a weight loss goal. Overall, monitoring your success is a crucial component of any weight loss program. It aids in keeping you inspired, responsible, and informed of your advancement, enabling you to make adjustments and acknowledge achievements along the route.

Chapter 3

Adding Healthy Habits to Your Lifestyle

*The Benefits of a Balanced Diet

Maintaining good health and preventing diseases require a balanced diet. It entails ingesting a range of various foods in the appropriate ratios to supply the body with the nutrients it requires to function correctly. Focus on including a variety of nutritional foods into your diet to support general health and weight management rather than limiting particular foods and food groups. Produce naturally has little fat and calories, but is nevertheless nutrient-dense and nourishing. The water and fiber it contains lend bulk to recipes. By substituting fruits and vegetables for components that have a greater caloric content, you may make delightful recipes that are lower in calories. A balanced diet consists of a variety of nutrients such as *fiber, vitamins, minerals, proteins, healthy fats, and carbohydrates*. Potassium, magnesium, and iron can assist to balance out sodium, which causes bloating. Leafy greens, the majority of "orange*" foods, sweet potatoes, melon, bananas, tomatoes, and cruciferous vegetables, notably cauliflower*, are foods high in nutrients to burn fats in the body. You may also assist in combating bloating by consuming low-fat dairy products, almonds, and seeds. They've also been connected to a slew of additional health advantages, including decreasing blood pressure, managing blood sugar, and lowering the risk of chronic illness in general. Each of these nutrients serves a particular purpose in the body, and a lack or overabundance of any one of them can cause a variety of medical issues. The majority of the calories we consume each day should come from carbohydrates because they are the body's main source of energy. Proteins are required for the healthy operation of the immune system as well as for the creation and repair of tissues. The brain, cell growth, and reduction of inflammation depend on healthy fats like omega-3 and omega-6 fatty acids. Although only in little levels, vitamins and minerals are essential for many body processes. Eating a meal that is balanced in nutrients and packed with fiber, protein, and healthy fats will alter your day, especially if you are presently skipping it and still finding it difficult to prioritize living a healthy lifestyle. By making you feel "overwhelmed" in the afternoon, skipping your major meal of the day may affect your hunger hormones later in the day, making it more difficult for you to resist overeating or seeking meals high in sugar and refined carbohydrates. Meals that will fill you up, keep you pleased, and ward off cravings later in the day are the greatest, heartiest meals. Make sure your morning meal has a source of lean protein, satisfying fat (*like eggs, unsweetened Greek yogurt, nuts, or nut butter), and fiber (like vegetables, fruit*, or 100% whole grains). Aim for a meal between 300 and 600 calories. You'll lose weight if you start your day with a nutritious mixture that stabilizes blood sugar. ***For instance, iron is necessary for producing healthy red blood cells, while vitamin C supports the immune system.*** Constipation can be avoided and maintained by eating enough fiber. It also aids in lowering the risk of diabetes, heart disease, and several types of cancer. A balanced diet can also aid in maintaining a healthy weight, lowering the risk of chronic illnesses like diabetes, heart disease, and some malignancies, and enhancing general health. For optimal health and well-being, a balanced diet is necessary. It entails consuming a range of foods in the correct quantities to give the body the nutrients it requires to operate as it should. We can enhance our general health and lower our risk of chronic illnesses by eating a balanced diet and choosing healthy food choices.

* macro- and micronutrients

For our bodies to function effectively, macronutrients and micronutrients are two categories of nutrients. We require greater amounts of macronutrients than micronutrients, which are needed in lesser proportions. ***Carbohydrates, proteins, and lipids are macronutrients***. Our bodies use proteins to build and repair tissues, as well as to produce enzymes and hormones, while carbohydrates are the main source of energy for our bodies. The storage of energy, insulation, and the absorption of several vitamins all depend on fats. ***Vitamins and minerals such as vitamin C, iron, and calcium are examples of micronutrients***. Vitamins are organic substances that our systems require in trace amounts for several processes, including energy metabolism, immune system health, and vision. On the other hand, minerals are inorganic chemicals that are crucial for hormone production, neuron function, and bone health. To meet our nutritional demands, a balanced diet that consists of a variety of nutrient-dense foods is crucial. Both macronutrients and micronutrients are required for sustaining good health.

foods that have undergone fermentation They improve the performance of beneficial bacteria while preventing the development of harmful germs. Probiotics are beneficial bacteria that are present in foods like sauerkraut, kimchi, kefir, yogurt, tempeh, and miso. Kimchi may offer anti-obesity properties, according to extensive research on the subject. Kefir may also aid in encouraging weight loss in overweight women, according to research. Prebiotic foods promote the development and activity of certain beneficial bacteria that help with weight management. Many fruits and vegetables, including chicory root, artichokes, onions, asparagus, leeks, and avocados, contain prebiotic fiber. Moreover, cereals like oats and barley contain it.

*Upholding a regular sleep schedule

For general health and well-being, it's critical to maintain healthy sleeping patterns. Even on weekends, try to keep your bedtime and wake-up times consistent. Establish a tranquil nighttime ritual that may involve a warm bath or shower, reading, or listening to soothing music. Ensure that it is cool, quiet, and dark in your bedroom. Get a cozy mattress and pillows. Electronic devices' blue light emissions have been shown to disrupt sleep. At least an hour before going to bed, try to avoid using computers, tablets, and phones. Alcohol and caffeine both have the potential to keep you awake. Before going to bed, stay away from these substances. Your sleep can get better if you exercise frequently. Just remember to finish your workout before going to bed. Sleep disturbances can be caused by stress. To relieve stress, try practicing relaxation strategies like meditation or deep breathing. You may enhance the quality of your sleep and feel more refreshed and invigorated throughout the day by using these suggestions.

*Reducing Stress

Stress is a normal aspect of life and can occasionally help us reach our goals by serving as a motivator. *But stress can have a detrimental effect on our physical and mental health, interpersonal relationships, and general quality of life when it becomes chronic or overwhelming. These are some* methods for controlling stress. Whether they are associated with *jobs, relationships, economics, health,* **or** *other areas*, it is critical to identify the sources of stress in our life. We can take action to decrease or manage the sources once we've identified them. Deep breathing, meditation, yoga, or progressive muscle relaxation are all relaxation techniques that can help lower stress levels and foster feelings of tranquility and relaxation. By releasing endorphins, enhancing mood, and fostering better sleep, regular exercise can assist to alleviate stress. Stress and overwhelm can result from bad time management. We can lower stress and boost productivity by setting priorities and making efficient use of our time. Speaking with friends, relatives, or a mental health expert can offer helpful support and aid with stress management. Keep in mind that stress management is a process that may need continual practice and effort. You may enhance your general well-being and quality of life by putting these techniques into practice and prioritizing stress management.

***Keeping tabs on your diet and exercise**

You can use tracking your diet and activity to help you reach your fitness and health objectives. select a tracking technique, You can track your meals and activity using a variety of applications and websites.

Fitbit, Lose It!, and MyFitnessPal are a few well-liked choices.

A spreadsheet or paper journal are other options. Establish attainable objectives, Before monitoring, it's crucial to establish reasonable objectives for oneself. Be specific in your goals and make sure they can be accomplished in a fair amount of time. It's crucial to track constantly if you want to receive the most accurate picture of your dietary consumption and exercise. Make it a routine to record your food and workouts each day. When keeping track of your diet and workout routine, it's critical to be honest with yourself as well. Never disregard meals or snacks or undervalue portion sizes. *Only if you use the information to make adjustments will tracking your diet and exercise be beneficial.* Find patterns in your eating and exercise behavior, then utilize that knowledge to modify your diet and exercise schedule. Remember that keeping track of your diet and activity is simply one tool you can use to achieve your fitness and health objectives. Prioritizing a healthy diet, consistent exercise, and sound sleep practices are crucial.

***Meal Preparation and Planning Advice.**

Maintaining a healthy and balanced diet requires the ability to plan and prepare meals. Make a week's worth of meals in advance. You can keep organized and make sure you have all the materials on hand by doing this. Don't forget to stock up on staples like rice, pasta, canned foods, spices, and herbs. It will be simpler to prepare meals on short notice as a result. Prepare a lot of food, and then put the leftovers in the refrigerator or freezer. You'll be able to prepare meals in the future with less time and effort thanks to this. Meals can be easily prepared in advance using slow cookers. You can prepare everything in the slow cooker in the morning and enjoy a hot meal when you get home. For a healthy diet, fresh fruits and vegetables are necessary. Eating spicy food can aid in calorie reduction. This is because the component capsaicin, which is present in both *jalapeno and cayenne which papers*, may raise your body's production of stress hormones like adrenaline, which can hasten the rate at which you burn calories. Also, consuming spicy peppers may encourage you to eat more slowly and limit your intake. You're more likely to remain aware of your hunger cues. Together with spicy peppers, ginger, and turmeric are other excellent options. When you can, try to include them in your meals. Create fresh dinners with leftover meats, vegetables, and grains. For instance, you can utilize leftover chicken to make a salad or a sandwich. Prepare items ahead of time by chopping veggies, marinating meats, and measuring them. When it comes to cooking, this will save you time. To eat healthily, you don't need to prepare elaborate meals. A few simple items can make delicious and healthful meals. The act of cooking ought to be joyful. Test out new dishes, play around with flavors, and take pleasure in the process.

Chapter 4

Workout to Lose Weight

* The Advantages of Exercise

Many advantages of exercise exist for both physical and mental health.
Exercise increases circulation, strengthens the heart and lungs, decreases blood pressure, and lowers risk factors for heart disease, stroke, and other cardiovascular issues. Exercise can enhance physical performance overall and promote flexibility while lowering the chance of injury. By

burning calories and boosting your metabolism, exercise can assist you in maintaining a healthy weight. Exercise releases endorphins, which enhance mood and general well-being while reducing stress, anxiety, and sadness. Frequent exercise will enhance your sleep, which will benefit both your physical and mental health. Exercise has been demonstrated to enhance cognitive abilities such as memory, focus, and judgment. The risk of chronic illnesses including diabetes, cancer, and osteoporosis can be reduced by exercise. Frequent exercise has been associated with a longer life expectancy and a lower risk of dying young. In general, exercise is necessary to keep one's health and well-being. Your physical and mental health, as well as your general quality of life, can be significantly improved by including regular physical activity in your daily routine. Adjustments to dietary habits and increased physical activity, usually in the form of exercise, are the least invasive weight loss strategies and those that are most frequently advised. The World Health Organization advises people to increase their physical activity while consuming fewer processed meals heavy in sugar, salt, and saturated fats. Long-term exercise regimens and anti-obesity drugs both reduce the amount of abdominal fat. Self-monitoring of nutrition, activity, and weight is a good way to lose weight, especially in the beginning stages of a program. According to research, persons who track their meals around three times per day and 20 times per month are more likely to lose clinically meaningful weight.

Maintaining a negative energy balance is what causes weight loss, not the kind of macronutrients (such as carbohydrates) that are ingested. Due to improved thermogenesis and satiety, high protein diets have demonstrated higher effectiveness for persons who eat whenever they want in the short term.

*Various Exercises for Losing Weight

Several different exercises might aid in weight loss.

workout for the heart: Your heart rate increases during this workout, which also burns calories. Examples include swimming, dancing, brisk walking, cycling, and running.

High-Intensity Interval Training (HIIT) is a type of exercise that involves short bursts of intensive activity followed by rest intervals or low-intensity exercise. It is a very efficient way to burn calories and may be done with bodyweight exercises or with the aid of machines like a treadmill or stationary cycle.

Strength training: Strength training can help you gain muscle, which can boost your metabolism and enable you to burn more calories even when you're not exercising. Examples include using resistance bands, lifting weights, and performing workouts with your body weight like pushups and squats.

Pilates: The core muscles are emphasized in this type of exercise, which also aims to increase flexibility and balance. By boosting muscle growth and boosting calorie expenditure, it can also aid in weight loss.

Yoga: Although it is not commonly thought of as a weight-reduction exercise, yoga can aid in weight loss by boosting strength, flexibility, and awareness. Some forms of yoga, such as power yoga, can also be highly physically taxing and can aid in calorie burning. Exercises are performed in succession, with little to no rest in between, during a circuit training session. By boosting muscle mass and burning calories, it can aid in weight loss. It's crucial to remember that combining diverse exercise types with healthy eating practices is the most efficient strategy to lose weight through exercise.

***Developing a Strategy for a Successful Workout**

A few essential steps go into developing an efficient fitness program:
Determine what you want to accomplish with exercise and set attainable, precise goals. Having a clear objective in mind will enable you to create a strategy that is customized to your requirements, whether it is for weight loss, muscle gain, or general fitness improvement.

Pick the right exercises: Choose workouts that are suitable for your current fitness level and that concentrate on the specific muscles you wish to strengthen. If you're unsure of what exercises to perform, talk to a personal trainer or rely on reliable fitness resources to help you make decisions.

Create a schedule: Allocate a regular time every day or week to exercise. To observe results and form a habit, consistency is essential.

Increase intensity gradually

When your fitness level rises, start with easier workouts and progressively make them harder. This will help you avoid harm and maintain your motivation as you make progress.

Include variation: Switch up your workouts to avoid getting bored and engage a range of muscles. Injuries and progress plateaus can both be avoided by doing this.

Observe your development:
Maintain a log of your workouts and advancement toward your objectives. This might assist you in determining where your plan needs to be modified or altered to continue moving forward. Discover ways to stay motivated, whether it be via exercising with a friend, enjoying music, or rewarding yourself when you achieve goals. The long-term success of your workout program depends on your ability to maintain motivation.

Chapter 5

Overcoming Plateaus and Stagnation

***Many factors can cause weight reduction to stagnate**

Your body adjusts to the lower calorie intake by slowing down your metabolism to save energy. Your weight reduction may slow down or possibly stop as a result of this.

Loss of Muscle: If you diet without exercising, you risk losing muscle mass in addition to fat. Your metabolic rate may be decreased as a result of slowing weight loss.

Water Retention: Your body may retain water for several causes, including hormonal changes, a high salt diet, or physical activity. This may give the impression that your progress has stopped even while your body's composition is shifting.

Inconsistent Calorie Intake: After a while of dieting, your body may have become accustomed to the calorie shortfall. You might need to lower your calorie consumption even more or up your exercise if you want to keep losing weight. Lack of sleep and stress can have an impact on your hormone levels, metabolism, and ability to control your eating. As a result, weight loss may become more difficult and may plateau. In general, weight reduction plateaus are typical, so it's crucial to maintain healthy routines and modify your diet and exercise program as necessary.

***How to break out of a rut**
It is claimed that progress in a certain area has reached a plateau when it has ceased or slowed down. Although learning plateaus are common, they can nevertheless be frustrating. You can keep moving forward by using the strategies listed below to overcome plateaus: The most frequent cause of plateaus is because you've become overly acclimated to your routine. By changing your habits, you can push yourself and promote new growth. Try to take a different tack on things, whether it entails reorganizing your to-do list or choosing a new tactic. It might be time to set a new goal if you've

been working toward the same one for a long time. Setting new goals can give you a sense of direction and aid in keeping your attention on the future. By using other people's input, you can identify areas where you need to improve. Be receptive to advice from people whose viewpoints you value and seek out. You can overcome a mental block by learning something new because it will provide your brain with new stimuli. Think about learning a new skill or registering for a course in a subject you've always been interested in. Even though plateaus may be disappointing, have a positive outlook. Remembering that progress takes time and effort, plateaus are a typical part of learning. By using these tactics, you can overcome growth and development obstacles in your chosen area.

Chapter 6

Loss Of weight and Supplements

*How Supplements Work Scientifically

Supplements are goods designed to provide extra nutrients, vitamins, minerals, herbs, or other substances to a person's diet that are thought to have health benefits. Depending on the exact supplement and the advantages claimed for it, the research behind supplements is complicated and varies. Generally speaking, a lot of supplements are based on a scientific study that has established the value of particular nutrients for health. Research has demonstrated, for instance, that vitamin D is crucial for bone health and may play a part in the immunological function. Not all supplements are supported by reliable scientific research. Several supplements are advertised with inflated promises and little to no evidence from science to back up their efficacy. Supplements can occasionally be dangerous if used in large doses or conjunction with specific drugs. It's crucial to understand that dietary supplements cannot take the place of a balanced diet and healthy lifestyle. Although certain people may benefit from specific supplements, they shouldn't be used as the major method of staying healthy. It's always important to see a healthcare professional before beginning any supplement regimen, especially if you take medication or have underlying health concerns.

***Herbs/Supplements for losing weight**

Garcinia Cambogia: This supplement is derived from the fruit rind of the Garcinia Cambogia plant. HCA is thought to stop the creation of fat and reduce appetite.

Green tea extract: This herb's catechins and caffeine are believed to speed up metabolism and help in fat burning.

raspberries: The chemical substances contained which are believed to boost metabolism and suppress appetite are used to make raspberry ketones.

Conjugated linoleic acid (CLA) is derived from the fatty acid present in meat and dairy products and is thought to promote muscle mass while decreasing body fat.

Forskolin: This substance, which is derived from the root of the Coleus plant, is thought to raise levels of the hormone cAMP, which speeds up metabolism and encourages fat loss. While there may be some evidence to support the usefulness of these Herb's supplements, it's critical to remember that they do not serve as a replacement for a balanced diet and regular exercise. Before beginning any new herb or supplement for weight loss programs, it is always advisable to speak with a healthcare expert.

*How to Choose Safe and Effective Supplements

Due to the supplement industry's lack of regulation and the prevalence of products with dubious safety and efficacy on the market, selecting safe and effective supplements can be difficult. But, there are certain actions you can do to improve your chances of selecting a supplement that is secure and efficient: A healthcare expert, such as a doctor, pharmacist, or qualified nutritionist, should be consulted before using any supplements. In addition to giving you advice on potential hazards and interactions with any medications or supplements you might be taking, they can assist you in determining whether a supplement is suitable for your health needs. Check for independent confirmation,   Inquire about dietary supplements that have been approved by independent   agencies   *like   NSF* International, ***ConsumerLab.com***, or the ***United   States   Pharmacopeia   (USP)***. These   organizations   evaluate supplements for purity, potency, and quality, and they can assist you in selecting supplements that adhere to strict guidelines. Check the ingredient and dosage information on supplement labels to make sure you are getting what you need. Look for products that include a list of the active substances' precise levels, as well as any additional compounds or additions that might be used. Avoid buying anything with dubious claims: Be cautious of supplements that make overly general or inflated claims or that guarantee miraculous outcomes. Since they are not designed to treat or cure any medical issues, supplements are not subject to the same regulations as pharmaceuticals. Choose supplements from well-known companies with a track record of making high-quality goods. Search for companies that have a solid track record among customers and healthcare professionals and have been around for a while. In general, it's wise to use caution while taking supplements and to do your homework before doing so. You can improve your chances of selecting secure and efficient supplements by working with a healthcare practitioner, looking for third-party verification, carefully reading labels, avoiding dubious promises, and selecting reliable brands.

Chapter 7

Modifying Your Lifestyle to Lose Weight

***Tips for long-term weight loss.**

The secret to reaching weight loss goals in a healthy and long-term way is to make permanent lifestyle adjustments. Establish attainable objectives, It's crucial to make goals that fit your lifestyle and are both attainable and realistic. Start with minor adjustments and gradually progress to more significant ones. A diet rich in fruits, vegetables, lean proteins, and whole grains should be the main focus. Steer clear of processed foods, sugary beverages, and a lot of saturated and trans fats. Ensure that you are adequately hydrated to lose weight and maintain good health. Try to consume eight glasses of water or more each day. Regular exercise should be a part of your regimen. Choose a habit-forming activity that you enjoy doing. Try to exercise for at least 30 minutes, most days of the week, at a moderate level. Make sure you are getting adequate rest because not getting enough sleep can also result in weight gain. Sleep for 7-9 hours every night. Weight gain and overeating are two effects of ongoing stress. Find healthy stress-reduction strategies, such as exercise, meditation, or time spent outside. Be consistent, When it comes to making long-lasting lifestyle changes, consistency is essential. Make good habits a part of your daily routine and maintain them. Be patient and gentle to yourself along the road, keeping in mind that losing weight is a journey. Although it takes time to adopt a sustainable lifestyle, the benefits are worthwhile.

***Stress management and emotional eating**

Slowing down to focus on things like the taste, textures, temperature, and smells of what you're eating can help with portion control. But emotional eating also means focusing on what you're eating and when this can help you identify unnecessary munching moments you may not realize you're engaging in throughout the day that may be tacking on extra calories. More importantly, try to avoid eating foods that you don't choose for yourself. Mindful eating can help shift the focus of control from external authorities and cues to your body's inner wisdom. Noticing where your extra calories come from is another step to making better choices in the short and long term. Although it can be challenging to manage stress and emotional eating, it is possible with the right tools. Finding the triggers is the first step in addressing stress or emotional eating. The most frequent causes were boredom, loneliness, anxiety, and depression. You can improve your self-awareness and lower your stress by practicing mindfulness, doing deep breathing exercises, or practicing meditation. This might help you recognize emotional depletion and direct you toward more effective coping skills. Your physical and mental health can be enhanced by eating a balanced diet. Always choose foods that are high in nutrients and low in sugar and unhealthy fats. If you're aware of the foods that are more likely to trigger emotional overeating in you, attempt to keep them away from your home and place of employment. Request support from friends and family, or consider meeting with a mental health professional. They can provide coping mechanisms and help with emotional eating and stress. Be aware that it can take some time to figure out what strategies for emotional eating and stress management work best for you. Be kind to yourself as you work to become a more positive, happier version of yourself.

Chapter 8

*Final thoughts and weight loss future steps

If you've been trying to lose weight, it's crucial to assess your success and make any required modifications. If you want to support your weight reduction objectives more effectively, take a look at your present eating behaviors and see if you can make any adjustments. If you want to lose weight, think about eating fewer calories overall, less processed food, and more lean protein, veggies, and fruits. A good weight loss strategy must include regular exercise as a key element. If you want to put more of a strain on your body, think about upping the quantity or intensity of your exercises or trying out new sports. Measure yourself frequently, keep track of your food consumption, and chart how much you exercise to keep track of your weight reduction progress. As a result, you'll be more driven to keep going and make any necessary changes. A licensed nutritionist or a personal trainer might be able to assist you in creating a plan that is specifically tailored to your requirements and way of life. ***Manage the emotional and psychological effects of weight reduction by joining a support group or consulting a therapist***. A thorough strategy that incorporates a nutritious diet, consistent exercise, and continuing support is needed to lose weight sustainably. These actions can help you move closer to your weight reduction objectives while also enhancing your general health and wellness.

*Resources for Supporting Weight Loss

There are numerous services available to help with weight loss success moving forward.

Here are some recommendations:

Support groups: Being a member of a group that promotes weight loss can provide you with accountability, inspiration, and a sense of belonging. *TOPS, Weight Watchers, and Overeaters Anonymous* are a few well-liked alternatives

Applications and websites: *You can track your progress, establish goals, and get advice and direction from a*

variety of apps and websites. SparkPeople, MyFitnessPal, and LoseIt! are a few well-liked choices. Working with a personal trainer or coach can offer you individualized advice and assistance that is catered to your unique requirements and goals.

Healthcare professionals: Speaking with a physician or certified nutritionist can be a great way to get advice and assistance for losing weight. Keep in mind that long-term weight loss is a journey, not a goal. You may maintain your motivation and accomplish long-term success by consistently looking for guidance and resources. Certain widely held notions about weight reduction have been demonstrated to either have less effect than generally thought or to be actively harmful. The notion that metabolism is the "key to weight" is "half reality and part myth," according to Harvard Health, since while metabolism does affect weight reduction, outside factors like nutrition and exercise have an equal impact. Fitness magazine diet plans are also frequently considered to be helpful but may be harmful by reducing daily consumption of necessary calories and nutrients, which can be hazardous depending on the individual and can be capable of discouraging people from trying to lose weight.

***Recap of important weight loss maintenance techniques**

Yes, let's review some effective methods for keeping off weight:

Regular exercise: Do physical activity five times a week for at least 30 minutes each session. Exercise is essential for weight management since it helps burn calories and preserve muscle mass.

Healthy eating: Have a varied diet that is high in fresh produce, whole grains, lean protein, and omega-3 fatty acids. Steer clear of processed foods, sugary beverages, and a lot of saturated and trans fats.

Portion control: Use smaller plates, measure your food, and forgo second helpings to keep track of portion sizes and reduce your calorie intake.

Eat mindfully by paying attention to your hunger and fullness signs and by taking your time and avoiding distractions. This encourages increased meal satisfaction and prevents overeating.

Self-monitoring: Keep tabs on your weight, activity, and food intake regularly to monitor your progress and make necessary modifications.

Support system: Surround yourself with individuals who are supportive of your efforts to lose weight and who promote healthy behaviors.

Consistency: Maintain healthy routines over time, even after achieving your weight loss objective. This supports weight loss maintenance and prevents weight gain.

Bonus contents

*List of the healthiest meals for weight loss

There isn't a single "magic" meal that can make you lose weight, but there are several items that, when added to a balanced diet, can help you achieve your weight reduction objectives. These are some foods that are frequently suggested for shedding pounds:

(Leafy greens) can make you feel full and satisfied since they are abundant in nutrients and low in calories.

(Whole grains) might make you feel fuller for longer since they include more fiber than processed grains.

(Lean protein source) These include meats like chicken, turkey, and fish as well as plant-based proteins like tofu, tempeh, and beans.

(Fruits and vegetables) are abundant in fiber, vitamins, and minerals while having few calories.

(Nuts and seeds) can make you feel full and satisfied since they are rich in fiber, protein, and healthy fats.

*(Low-fat dairy products)*maybee a healthy source of protein and calcium, but be careful to pick low-fat varieties to limit your calorie intake.

(Avocado) Although having a lot of calories, avocados are a fantastic source of fiber and healthy fats, which may make you feel satiated and full. Keep in mind that achieving a calorie deficit by burning more calories than you take in is the key to losing weight. Including these items in a nutritious, balanced diet can boost your efforts to lose weight.